LIVING YOUR DIFFERENCE

---

3 POWER MOVES—TO KICK START YOUR
MENTAL SUCCESS

JOSEPH MICHAEL DOSS

CONTENTS

THE BIRTH

As I begin this chapter, I want to say that I think everyone has the ability to change their life for the better. Every person has the right to live the life they desire and to feel good about themselves. My journey of self-discovery and coming into a beautiful and wonderful life is one of uniqueness. I want to paint a vivid picture of the beginning of my life. It began as a life with limitations, but with the help of others, you will see that I was able to break out of that box of limitations.

My name is Joseph Michael Doss, and if you could take a glimpse at me through this book right now, you would see a young man who can breathe, talk, and even dance a little. I presently can do all these things without struggle, but this wasn't always so. You see, I came into this world much earlier than anyone expected —twenty-four weeks old, weighing only one pound and seven ounces. Because of this early entrance, I dealt with some life-threatening challenges that I had no control over. If you look at the picture in the back of the book, you will see a mini mini-me, so small that my father was able to hold me in the palm of his hand.

My premature birth brought many challenges for me, my parents, and the doctors. I had bleeding in my brain that the doctors indicated may have happened as my mom's body pushed me out. There wasn't really anything they could do to stop the bleeding except to take a wait-and-see approach and let the brain heal on its own. After about two days, the bleeding stopped. My lungs were pretty small and needed help to work consistently, so I was connected to a lung machine that helped me breathe. To keep my heart pumping steadily, I was also attached to a machine that stimulated my heart to make sure it did not stop pumping. A major situation occurred when my intestines perforated inside my body. Now the question on everyone's mind was

. . . Will Joseph live or die?

When the doctors informed my parents that I needed emergency surgery to fix my intestines, they also explained that they needed to clean out the intestines that were perforated. However, it was crucial that a particular valve be present so the intestines could grow again. If this important valve was damaged or missing, I would not be able to continue to live. My parents told me they prayed and believed that whatever was necessary to be present would be in place, and it was. The surgery was very successful, and I began to develop and grow new intestines.

I was in the NICU (Neonatal Intensive Care Unit) from October 1997 to April 1998, fighting for my life. Because I was so small and now out of the womb, I needed to be in the NICU in an incubator until my body developed and got stronger. I could not go home until I was in a stable condition. This growth process required six months of living in an incubator box.

The incubator provided a controlled environment of care and protection for me. Mom would come in the mornings, and the nurses would let her take me out of the incubator box and wrap me up. She would hold me on her chest for hours, singing and talking with me. Dad would come at night and take me out, hold me, and talk with me.

Every day for six months, Mom and Dad came to the hospital. Some days were a struggle because if my body wasn't in a stable condition, or if I had a fever or an elevated heart rate, Mom wasn't allowed to take me out to hold me; instead she could only sit close to the incubator where she would sing and talk to me through the opening.

When I think about my parents, I think about how they didn't give up and stayed strong throughout this time. What is so unique about my mom is that as an Early Childhood Educator, she was knowledgeable about the developing child. When she found herself in the position of having a son so early, she decided not to let what was happening to her and me defeat her.

Even though there were some moments of fear, my mom stayed positive, and that's how she overcame the fear. She told me that the tough times were times when she just totally depended on her faith in God. My Dad, who is a 6-foot-4inches-tall, muscular man, who by occupation is an amazing electrician, told me that my premature birth was tough for him. He said that at first, he couldn't understand why things were happening the way they were. But he knew he needed to be strong for me. My parents were a comfort for each other and believed that I would get better each day . . . and I did.

Around the month of March, the hospital informed my parents that I could go home in April. I was developing as well as could be expected. I was stable enough to leave the hospital, but I needed some assistance, so I left the hospital with three monitoring machines: for my heart, my lungs, and my brain. As each day went by, I began to get stronger. Mom took good care of me and monitored all of the machines. By June 1998, I was off all the machines, developing and growing, but I still had to continue to be monitored because I began to have some seizures. Thanks to the care of a loving and strong family, I was able to overcome.

My life began with some major challenges, but my family was there to support me. I realize now how important it is to have family support. I was in an encouraging and supportive family as I grew. I was getting Early Childhood Development Services to help with speech and physical and occupational development.

As a growing child, I was happy. I loved to meet people. I loved to play. I went to sleep happy, I woke up happy. As a kid, I remember playing basketball outside with my brothers, who were very competitive about winning. My oldest brother, Jonathan, was always the one who would get the ball and shoot it in the basket from behind the free-throw line. We called him the shooter. My next oldest brother, Joshua, was fast and would dribble the ball and drive it to the basket. We called Joshua the driver.

My youngest brother, Jordan, was a combination of both of them. Jordan would sometimes shoot from a long distance and then sometimes he would drive it to the basket. I was just happy to be out there playing with them. Because of some developmental challenges, I didn't run as fast as Jonathan or drive to the basket like Joshua, but I would sometimes beat them to the spot where they were shooting and block the ball. Once I blocked the ball, I would turn around and shoot it toward the basket. I was strong and determined whether I succeeded or not, but when I did make the shot, my brothers and parents would cheer for me.

My family would always say, "Joseph, you are very persistent."

My brothers always included me. My life at home was fun with my parents and brothers.

When Mom enrolled me in the local public elementary school, the environment was very new and scary for me. My loving and caring family was not with me in the mornings anymore, leaving me to face uncomfortable, unkind, and unexpected situations on my own. I expected to have just as much fun as I did with my family, but I found out that kids are not so nice if you are premature.

2

———

ELEMENTARY SCHOOL

When I turned five, I entered the local elementary school and things changed. In this chapter, you will see that my life took a turn; a turn that would last a very long time. This part of my life was a time I didn't readily talk about, but through self-discovery, I have conquered those thoughts and want to share my story. Let's see what happened.

When I was in grades Kindergarten to fourth, I found out that not everyone was as happy as I was, and that the kids could be really, really mean. Kids did not want to play with me; they would laugh at me and use hurtful words. One kid told me he didn't like the way I talked. At the time, I was receiving speech therapy and struggling with the pronunciation of my words. Instead of being understanding and tolerant, they were mean.

I remember going home and asking Mom, "Why are the kids so mean? Why do kids feel like they can say cruel things? I am a kid just like they are!"

Mom sat me down and said, "Son, listen to me, you did not come into this world like the average person, you had a special birth because you are a very special person. You are different and that is okay. Some of the things you do, and the way you act, the kids won't understand because they want you to act like them, but you are not like them, and that's okay." Then she said, "Joseph, I love you just the way you are."

The kids saw me as socially awkward because of the way I talked, because of the way I walked (I walked on my toes), and because I related to the teachers more than they did. They called me the teacher's pet, but the teachers understood me. For a long period of time, I kept doubting what my mom was saying to me. I would think to myself that Mom was wrong and the kids were right. I really did want to be part of the kid group.

When I started fifth grade, school got worse and even brutal. I just wanted to be accepted by the kids even though they were saying things like, "Joseph you are ugly, you are weird, and you are too tall to play." I thought what they said was right because I kept hearing it every day. I cried all the time. If school was going to be like this, I didn't want to go to school anymore. I was picked last for group projects. The teacher had to make the children pick me (that was really sad).

During gym class, none of the guys picked me to be on their basketball team. I thought to myself, *It isn't fair that these kids don't like me.* I was a fun person, my brothers had a good time with me, and my mom was always laughing at my jokes and encouraging me to sing, even though I really could not carry a note. I thought to myself, *What is wrong with these kids?*

As I got older, my mom kept saying, "Joseph, it's okay, it's okay, it's okay."

My mom began working with me on what was special about me. She gave me a book to read, entitled *Think Big* by Nancy Carlson. She began to highlight my strengths and celebrate the great things about me.

Even though I was hearing Mom, I still had to go back to that elementary school where I was crying and sad. I wrote a letter to a girl I liked, and she threw it in the garbage can right in front of me without reading it. I got the courage to tell a girl how much I liked her, and she told me that she did not like me because I was ugly. I bought gifts for girls on Valentine's Day (against Mom's wishes) so they would like me. They took my gifts, but they still didn't talk to me after Valentine's day. There were two students I did call my friends: Sam and Julian. They were boys who didn't care about what the other kids thought of me and befriended me anyway. Julian invited me to his birthday parties, and Sam would play basketball with me at the end of school while we were waiting for our parents to pick us up.

In sixth grade, my life began to change. This change happened the day Ms. G became my teacher. Now let me tell you about Ms. G. She was in her thirties and not very tall; she stood about 4 feet 9 inches. She always wore high heels and had beautiful blonde hair. She presented herself with a strong confidence I admired.

I wanted to be confident like her. She was my favorite teacher. She befriended me and allowed me to share with her my struggles. She treated me kindly and told me that I didn't need to fit in. What she said sounded like what Mom was saying.

Ms. G was a big part of my self-discovery. Before she came, I felt like I didn't have anyone to talk to. Although I did not see it at the time, she made herself available to me always. She was the person at the elementary school that I could come and talk with about anything. She would give me advice, but she would also just listen to me. She made me feel like I belonged when everyone else was treating me like an outcast.

Ms. G began to work with me on self - confidence and helping me see the good qualities I possessed. Not only was she a great teacher, but she was my best friend. She taught me life lessons. One of those lessons was how to ignore what the kids said or thought about me. Not only did she teach me this lesson, but she also demonstrated it to me, training me by example. I would observe Ms. G as she interacted with other adults and how she demonstrated confidence while working with them. It didn't really matter to her what they thought about her, whatever she wanted to accomplish, she did. She helped me overcome the fear of what people thought about me and challenged me in my thinking.

Ms. G. would always say something to me that made me laugh. I was very happy to hear this statement. She would say, "There's nobody like Joseph Doss, and there will never be another one like him." The thought, the fact that someone at the school took the time to think about me in a positive way, and actually shared it with me, was amazing. I began to discover myself, but you must remember, I was still in my pre-teen years, and that box of peer pressure was still there.

I was in eighth grade, getting ready to go to high school, when I met Mr. J, our part-time recess monitor who taught me how to play chess during recess. He was a young man who had just graduated from high school and was now in college. I literally looked up to him because he was very tall, about 6 feet 2 inches, and he had a strong and fit body. He taught me strategies in thinking and helped me become a good chess player. We were talking one day about some of the struggles I was experiencing with the kids, and he said something that will always stick with me for life: "Joseph, don't worry about the kids in this school because you are going to high school and it will get better."

After hearing what Mr. J said, I had high hopes for high school. I thought it would get better, but it only got worse. I wondered if Mr. J knew that these high schoolers were just like the kids at the elementary school, just a bit older. Did he really understand the truth and perhaps didn't want to tell me? This puzzled me.

———

3

HIGHS & LOWS OF HIGH SCHOOL

In this chapter, you will see how all of my expectations for high school came crashing down. In the midst of my high school crisis, three special teachers came into my life and gave me some things I needed to continue on my journey of self-discovery. These teachers were very honest with me, and they gave me the freedom to be me.

The first two years of high school were really tough. During the last two years of high school, a shift took place in my life. By the time I left high school, I was comfortable in my own skin. Things had turned around for me. I was helping other kids break out of this peer-pressure box, this box that makes kids feel they aren't good enough and that they won't succeed unless they do it the way everybody else does it. I was realizing that this might be the special thing that I was meant to do in life. Come, let's hear about my high school journey...

When I walked into this new big building, I was excited. I was thinking to myself, yes, this is high school—a new beginning and a fresh start. I will have new friends even though I see some of the kids from my old elementary school in attendance. There were lots and lots of kids; surely I would make some friends, or so I thought.

Every student was a part of a class called "Advisory," which was supposed to be an information class. The teacher would take attendance and share important school information. We were able to do homework and then, for the rest of the period, we could visit with friends. Well, this was a class I really did not like.

There were groups of students who

would sit together, and their whole purpose during this time was to make jokes about me. I would laugh, too, because I thought maybe if I laughed at myself, it wouldn't hurt so much, but it still hurt.

The beginning of high school was not good. I began to feel those same feelings I had in elementary school of not belonging. Some things the students would say or talk about I did not readily pick up on. It took me a little extra time to think about the things they would say, but I guess my information-processing speed was not fast enough for them. Some of the kids would say, "Joseph you didn't get that. Man, you are a little slow."

It wasn't enough that I was struggling with the students and trying to fit into this peer-pressure box, the box that made me feel like I wasn't good enough and that I wouldn't succeed in life unless I did it like everybody else, but unfortunately, I had teachers who listened to the kids and displayed to me through their attitudes that they didn't like me, and that really hurt. I just could not comprehend or accept teachers acting like the kids.

Even though I wasn't being treated right, I had such a desire to help other kids that were getting treated like me or worse. It seemed like they couldn't handle it, and maybe they didn't have other people in their lives helping them, or a strong family support system. I really wanted to help. I wanted to be the voice of the kids being taken advantage of in some capacity. I did not want them to be left out.

The high school dances were torturous. Wanting to connect with the kids, I would go to these dances even though Mom would say, "Joseph, I don't understand why you want to put yourself in an uncomfortable situation. You don't have to go to this dance."

I didn't really know why either, except that I had hope that maybe things would change. No change occurred. When I arrived, the kids acted toward me like they always did—like I didn't exist.

The school provided the kids with a

picture booth at the dance. Everyone was taking turns going into the booth to take pictures together. Since I was not part of the cool group, no one took pictures with me. I stood by the booth, hoping to take some pictures with someone. Some of the kids felt sorry for me and decided to ask me to take pictures. When they asked if I wanted to take a picture, I would readily say yes. Now, I laugh about being so desperate, but back then, it was not so funny.

I always tried "keeping up with the Joneses" but the Joneses were always changing for me. For example, one time I was in the gym, and all the boys were shooting from the three-point line. Sometimes they would make it, and when they did, the kids sitting in the gym would cheer and clap for them. I thought maybe if I did the same thing, I would get the same response.

I had been working on this shot with my brothers. When I began to hit a good amount of shots from the three-point line, the kids in the gym looked surprised.

They were not cheering and clapping for me; they actually began to leave the gym. They looked at me as if I was weird. This taught me a very important lesson: the rules of engaging with these kids were different for me. It wasn't what I did, it was who I was. It was Joe Doss shooting those shots, and "he is the one we are not supposed to like." So, if the kids didn't like me, I wasn't going to receive any approval from them. The word that went around was "stay away from Joe Doss."

What I really hated in high school was that I would be speaking with someone, when another person would come up and interrupt my conversation and be very rude about it. This demeaning behavior was very insulting and made me think small about myself. I began to think about my life and whether I wanted to continue to be treated like this. I thought maybe it would be better if I didn't exist.

4

———

THE TURNAROUND

My junior year came, and Mr. W became my Advisory teacher. Mr. H was my English teacher and Mr. N was my Humanities teacher. What a wonderful year! I felt God was smiling at me. (God was probably always smiling, I just wasn't tuned in or aware.)

Mr. W was not only my Advisory teacher, but he was also my Gym teacher. Mr. W was not a tall or short man. He was of medium build and very muscular. He worked out in the gym every day before school and he always, I mean always, wore sweatpants. He wore sweatpants to every event. If we had a dress-up day, he was in sweatpants. If he was meeting with important people in the building, he wore sweatpants.

Mr. W realized how the kids were treating me, and he said to me, "Joe Doss, I want you to be the leader that you are." So he put me in a leadership position as the Speaker of the class. I would receive the information for the class and make the announcements. The kids now had to listen to me.

Mr. H, my English teacher, was a family man. His family was very important to him. He spoke about his family all the time. His kids and wife were very special to him. He would ask me about my family and inquired about my mom and dad's parenting style, and then he would tell me how he and his wife were parenting their children.

In the classroom, Mr. H gave me the freedom to be me. One day in our English class, he gave me the opportunity to be the teacher for the day. He always drilled into my head this one thing: "Joseph, people are always going to judge you, but don't let that phase you because people are going to talk about you your whole life, but what you need to do is rise above that. The way you do that is to stay focused on what you are doing and don't focus on what anyone else is doing."

Mr. N was a man who was about 5 feet 7 inches tall. He was very energetic and determined. He was knowledgeable about all subjects in life. He always wanted to share his knowledge. He would always tell me what he thought was true about a situation and would not sugarcoat the information. Mr. N was the teacher who really solidified this whole topic of acceptance for me and helped me become the person I am today.

He gave me a platform that wasn't offered to the other students even though he had an opportunity to offer it to them. Other students wanted this platform, but he gave it to me. What Mr. N did was introduce me to part of my future. I became the host of the school Variety

Show, Culture Fest Show, and any other show we had. This was really big for me. I asked Mr. N why he chose me, and he said, "Because you are the one and only Joe Doss."

After doing a pretty good job of hosting the shows and hearing what Mr. N said, my confidence soared. Now knowing that I was "The one and only Joe Doss," the message of "Stay away from Joe Doss" did not matter to me at all.

Having these three amazing teachers speak (and continue to speak) into my life made the sounds and talk of the kids very small. I began to see the kids in a different light. They were hurting being caught up in this peer-pressure box, the box that made them feel like they weren't good enough, and in order to succeed in life, they would have to do it like everybody else.

There was a girl named Kelly, whom I really didn't know personally, but she sought me out for some advice. Kelly was a popular girl with a lot of friends. She was in a toxic relationship with her friends, and she didn't know how to get out of it.

She didn't know how to get out of it. She struggled with whether she really should get new friends, and if she did proceed with acquiring new friends, what would her old friends think? I told her to think about how her friends make her feel, and if it is not a good feeling, is she okay with that? If after she thinks about how her friends make her feel, and she is not okay with that, then she needs to decide to move on with new and positive friends.

I told her what my teachers told me, and that was that she needed to value herself over any other person because her mental health was more important than anything. I'd hoped Kelly would take my advice, but I didn't see her after that encounter.

The wonderful and outstanding teachers who knew me, and whom I trusted, always gave me advice that helped me grow strong mentally. Some of the things I enjoyed about their partnership were that they honestly and genuinely cared about me. They saw me for who I really was, which is why I liked them.

Overall, high school had a huge impact on my life. I learned a lot. The most important thing I learned was to always stay true to myself. I shifted my thinking to become a person that knows I am good enough—more than good enough. I know that I don't have to do it like everyone else in order to succeed. I am out of that BOX. Now, let's figure out your particular box that you may be in. Let's find out what is keeping you inside and limiting your full potential, and let's overcome it.

If you are ready to make a change, continue reading. In this next chapter, I would like to help you work at becoming authentically you.

———

5

THREE STEPS TO FREEDOM

In today's world, the majority of people are trying to fit in. When is the last time you've gone without wondering what somebody thought about you, or thinking that you are not enough, or sensing that you are not really being true to yourself?

Some of us are living dreams that others desire for us. Through my own self-discovery, I learned how to become aware of my unique self. I have been able to identify and discover my difference, and I want to help you do the same. Your difference is what makes you uniquely you, and your difference is what will keep you relevant. If we were all the same, life would be quite boring.

My life experience and unique point of view allow me to be credible. If you are ready to get the things in life that you desire, and develop the special relationships that have escaped you, then it is time to start thinking outside the box. You can live in your true self. You can love "you" every single day of every single week. You can be proud of the person you are.

Even when the odds are against you, you can still win. You can always get out of the box—the box that makes you feel you aren't good enough, and that makes you feel like you won't be successful if you don't do what everybody else is doing. Let's talk about being the best version of you and finally getting out of your BOX.

The way you think is not wrong, (no judgment) you just don't have another way to think. My three steps (power moves), will bring freedom to your life.

Following these steps will help you become the real you. You will change your life for the better by changing your thinking. Know this: everything in your life starts with a thought.

I get that you feel alone and that nobody cares. I get it because I have walked in the same shoes, but this is why you must become aware of what you are thinking.

Let's look at my story. I started out this life in an incubator box, but not only was I in an incubator box physically, but when I began my schooling, I was mentally in an incubator box trying to be accepted by the kids. My thoughts of being accepted, and the limiting thoughts I embraced, would not allow me to become aware of what was good about me.

Step One

Becoming aware is very necessary because we operate in life on autopilot. You have developed habits and beliefs that guide your life without you even thinking about them. When you want to make changes, it can only happen by first having the thought of change and then thinking about the process it will take to change.

Becoming aware of your thoughts, and taking time on purpose to ponder and reflect on what you are thinking, is a form of meditation. You have to begin meditating on positive thoughts and not negative. If you change your thoughts, you can change your life.

Capture your thoughts.

You say, "how can I do that?"

You can only do that by choosing what thoughts to think. A bird flies over your head, but you do not let him make a nest, and so the same is true with your thoughts. Research shows that we have 2,500–3,300 thoughts every hour, and it is impossible to take all of them in. You get to choose which thoughts you want to think. So choose the good ones that will begin to shift your life from negative to positive.

After you have become aware of your thoughts and begin to choose positive thoughts about your life and your future, you want to write down what you are thinking. I call this action *Writing your Life Vision*.

Your Life Vision could be a dream, a goal, an objective, a mission, or your values. It is personal to you, but you must be willing to do the work necessary to make it happen. Now I know that people say all the time to write things down, and usually, we don't follow that instruction, but if we did, we would see that it really works.

What happens when you write it down, put it on paper, make a vision board, journal your thoughts, or type on your smartphone? I will tell you what happens. Your thoughts are going from your mind to the paper. Your brain is stimulated when you engage in these activities. By doing such activities, you begin to see more clearly what you are thinking and begin to visualize your future life. Writing it down or getting it in front of you makes you look at it differently, and when you see it physically, you begin to see it in your mind's eye—your imagination.

I have actually engaged in this process and been successful. Thoughts I have about my life and things I desire for my future, I have put on a vision board. This board represents my future. I have pictures of places I want to visit. I have written goals of becoming a bestselling author and becoming an impactful public speaker.

This vision board is positioned in a place where I can look at it at least five times a day. I have a smaller vision card that I carry with me. One of the goals I set for myself was to lose twenty pounds in forty five days as I was getting ready for a wedding. Seeing that goal as much as I did, inspired me to take action. I changed my diet and worked out three times a week with a trainer. I actually lost over twenty pounds and have maintained the new weight.

You want to look at what you wrote at least three times a day. What is this doing? This is giving you an image of what you desire. This image brings you closer to your goal because you have now begun to focus and see yourself attaining it. Understand that anything you focus on expands and will show up in your life.

Now that you are choosing to think positive thoughts for your life, and you have taken action to write it down so that you can keep focusing on the good you desire for your life, you must take note of what you are saying.

What you say must agree with what you are thinking and seeing in your imagination and with what you have written down.

There are several ways we communicate in life, but one very important way is through the vehicle of words. Your words are very important. How important are your words? They can make or break your future and the future of others. Words connect us to each other. When you choose to give out negative words, or receive negative words, a bad connection is made, and then you experience negative emotions. Once this negative connection is made, you are going to have to counter it with a positive connection using positive words. Studies show that there is an optimal ratio of five positive comments to offset one negative comment. We want to always be saying positive words, and then we won't have to offset the negative words. Remember the power of your words.

If you would take an honest look at the things you say throughout the day to yourself, you will see that you are probably not saying positive things. Imagine what would happen if other people could hear your inner dialogue. The things you say are probably about things you are worried about, concerned about, or you may even be saying to yourself that good things won't happen for you.

When you are engaged in this process of self-talk, it can be negative talk or positive talk, but this activity of self-talk actually determines your life.

In my story about my school experience, kids were saying negative things about me. Remember how I began to say those negative things about myself and was doubting the positive talk my mom was saying to me? This kept me in a negative box. The negative self-talk I engaged in was critical, self-defeating, painful, and depressing.

It wasn't until I started to believe and started saying the positive things that my mother and my teachers said about me that I got out of that negative low self-esteem box. Using positive self-talk is a powerful tool. It increased my self-confidence and curbed the negative emotions I was experiencing.

Self-talk is the most powerful talk you can engage in because this is the talk that comes from your inner voice. I define the inner voice as an integrated pattern of thoughts, and these thoughts turn into a dialogue of what you think and believe. From this dialogue, you take action and make decisions in your everyday life. The things you say in self-talk are what you really believe—whether it is positive or negative.

Because self-talk is so powerful, make sure that when you engage in self-talk, that it is positive. The words you say to yourself need to elevate to positive words. Get rid of the negative words and replace them with positive words. I know you might want to say something negative, but that isn't what you really want to happen. Your results will be far better by saying the positive things you want. If you begin to speak what you want, (the positive things) you will begin to see it, and then it has no option but to be reproduced in your life.

You are unique because of the specific qualities you possess. Discovering what your unique qualities are, and then speaking them to yourself, will build up your confidence.

No one will be able to build up your confidence but you. When you have strong confidence in yourself, you begin to love yourself, and with self-love, you are powerful.

Say words that are empowering and positive. If your self-talk is negative, look yourself in the mirror and ask yourself, "Am I being who I truly am? Am I loving myself?" If the answer to these questions is no, then change what you are saying about yourself.

Now, when you begin this process, it will seem like nothing is happening, but changes in life happen over time. You will determine whether it will be a short time or a long time by the frequency of the effort you put into it.

Whether you repeat it to yourself three times a day or once a month, you will determine the results. Be a proactive person. The authentic self that you want to be in your life will appear as you continue this process. You will exceed your own expectations and abundantly receive the rewards of your thoughts. Make up your mind to do something different by taking these Three Steps of Freedom. Enjoy the new life you will experience—the new life you will create. You no longer have to be bound by what people say.

6

———

RAISING HOPE

Where you are in your life today has a lot to do with the choices you have made. When I decided to listen to and believe the people who were positive in my life, my life began to change. There is someone who is speaking in your life who is positive. Cut out the negative sounds and the negative self-talk. Begin the Three Steps of Freedom, which will take you outside of the box of limitations. Listen to the encouraging and positive words from your own self-talk and from others. Watch what happens.

Your core beliefs are going to play a significant role in how you take action.

Don't continue to fit into a box you don't belong in. When you are operating in your authentic self, you'll see how many amazing things will happen and how many awesome opportunities will present themselves.

I promise, if you receive the message relayed in this book and decide to apply it to your life, you will get out of your box of limitations and begin living free. You will be able to recognize what is holding you back and then possibly be able to help others who might be struggling through the exact same thing. Don't be the person who misses out on their dream.

Get Out Of Your Box!!!

ACKNOWLEDGMENTS

Every teacher has go-to catchphrases meant to give solace to students and parents in times of doubt. I've been a teacher for almost fifteen years. I have two favorites, both of which were shared with me by my father. Dad heard them from his teachers. These bits of wisdom are time tested. First, everybody is a package of strengths and weaknesses; and second, different flowers blossom at different times. Everyone has strengths. Figuring out your strengths and how to use them to your advantage is everyone's challenge. Everyone has weaknesses.

Figuring out how to mitigate them; how to prevent them from impeding your goals is also a challenge we all must face. It is as difficult to engage in the kind of self-discovery to truly access one's own strengths as to confront one's own weaknesses. For some, it is more difficult than others, thus the truism that different flowers blossom at different times.

There is presumed beauty and strength in all of our beings. Despite that, individuals can grow frustrated with themselves. When will it actualize into self-confidence and self-reliance? How much can anyone control the process? The experience of growing into yourself is unique to all people, and some are more aware and reflective of the process as a whole. When you have a concept of the world around you, the people in it, the rules (written and not) that govern relationships, your own dreams, and your own strengths, then you can exercise some control of your fate. Or, you can say forget all of that, and assert yourself anytime you're ready.

This is where one of my heroes comes into the picture. He is a hero because he lives life with a simple lesson in mind, and we could all stand to learn the Joe Doss lesson: people should be their best selves instead of trying to fit in a mold. If you live as your best self, then the next day you might even be better. When

Joe came to high school, he was just beginning to discover his strengths and weaknesses. In the beginning, he struggled with caring about what other people thought, but through some inner work, he began to be his best self every day. Joe began to be committed to being himself, and let others come to appreciate him. Joe went from wanting to be in the group to becoming a leader; even if he didn't have an army. He came to class ready to work and push others to do the same.

When Joe began to blossom, his work ethic would be augmented by dissatisfaction with anything short of his own high standards that he set for himself. He frequently asked how he could improve and sought a deeper understanding of the topics he studied. Joseph began to make creative connections and draw impressive conclusions from class to life. It was exciting to watch Joseph come into his unique self.

Joseph is a personable young man. Joe was the Master of Ceremonies for the high school Annual Variety Show. I knew his confidence, good nature, and sense of humor made him the perfect man for the job. It required flexibility and poise. He didn't let me down. It was his responsibility to keep eight hundred of his schoolmates entertained and in good spirits while the tech crew resolved problems. He was perfect, and I was very proud of him.

This is the Joe Doss I know. He was a young man in high school, who came not quite sure of himself, trying to figure out this social scene, but didn't quite know himself. He began to know the world as he sought to understand himself and in doing so, his place in the world revealed itself. Now, Joseph (Mr. Doss) is authoring a book. Joe was a role model for the people in his life when he was in high school, and he's a role model now. I can only imagine the impact this book can have on the people who read it. This book is a true extension of Joe; its goodness will not have to work too hard to impact you, and frankly, if this book doesn't impress upon you, it might not be the book's fault.

— ZACKARY NOVAK

Inspiration, it must be humbly admitted, often owes its genesis to the most persistent of us. Rocky ran the stairs, Achilles braved the Trojan force and David stood his ground at the feet of a giant. And whether on purpose or by chance, the persistent seem never to fail in inspiring us. Joseph; an idol of persistence, inspires us in ways one could only imagine from a character in a book would. An inability to give up on life, fostered at birth, has carried his morale through time itself. This story, his story, is not only a story of ups and downs, chuckles and tears, good times and bad times, but it is a story of persistence. A story that speaks to the seemingly forgotten, the painfully mistreated, the way too-early bloomers, the late developers, and the ones who have been told that *they might make it*. And who better to tell this story; than

Joseph, a man who has been told from the early stages of his gestation...*that he would not make it*.

— Joshua Doss

Loving, fearless, generous, resilient, self-assured. These are just a handful of the adjectives that describe Joseph Michael Doss. Joseph and I met in 2008, and little did I know what a profound influence we would have on each other.

Throughout the past decade, Joseph faced many challenges, both academically and socially.

Reading and math were a struggle. Peers were not always kind or inclusive. Many people would let these difficult experiences create doubt, make them bitter, or even give up, but not Joseph. Instead, he used them to ignite a drive to become a man who is true to himself and always kind to others.

One of my life's happiest moments was attending Joseph's high school graduation ceremony. I knew this was just the beginning of a life that would make this world a better place. While I have no children of my own, I take deep pride in his accomplishments. Joseph's spirit shines so brightly that anyone who meets him is made better.

When Joseph told me that he was writing a book, my heart burst with pride. So when he asked me to write this, I was overwhelmed and honored. I knew it was one of the important tasks that I would do in my life. He has inspired me to always look for the positive in any situation and be the best I can be. I look forward to seeing what life holds in store for him.

— STACY G.

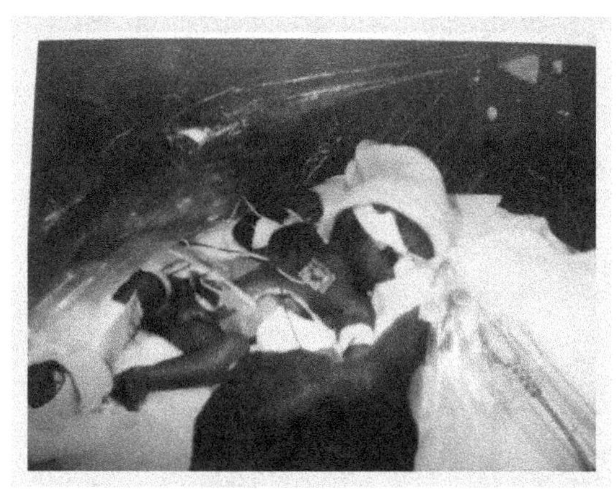

Joseph Michael Doss, seven hours old,

1lb. 7 oz

ABOUT THE AUTHOR

"Live Your Best Life."

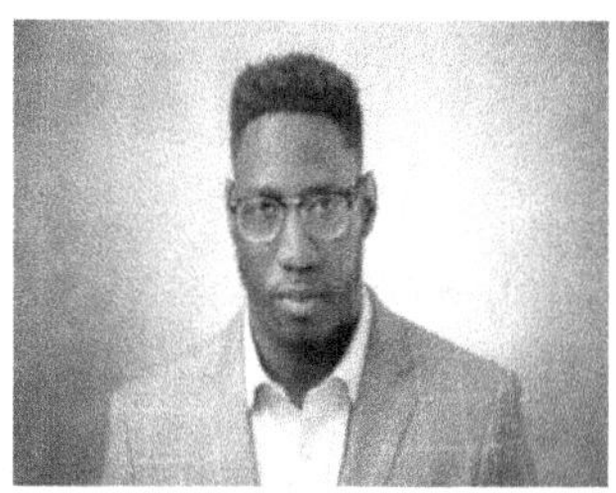

Joseph Michael Doss is a new author with a passion for helping people overcome life's limitations. He is a brother of four, a Public Speaker and Entrepreneur.
Joseph recalls the pain and struggle of his School Life. Through Self-Discovery and some special teachers, along with family support, he was able to turn it around.

Joseph believes that everybody deserves to live the life they desire. His book gives the reader some strategies to make this happen. When we proceed to live our best life, we make the world a better place.

Joseph is available for Speaking Engagements.

<u>Contact Information:</u>

Joseph Michael Doss

Email: JosephMDoss18@gmail.com

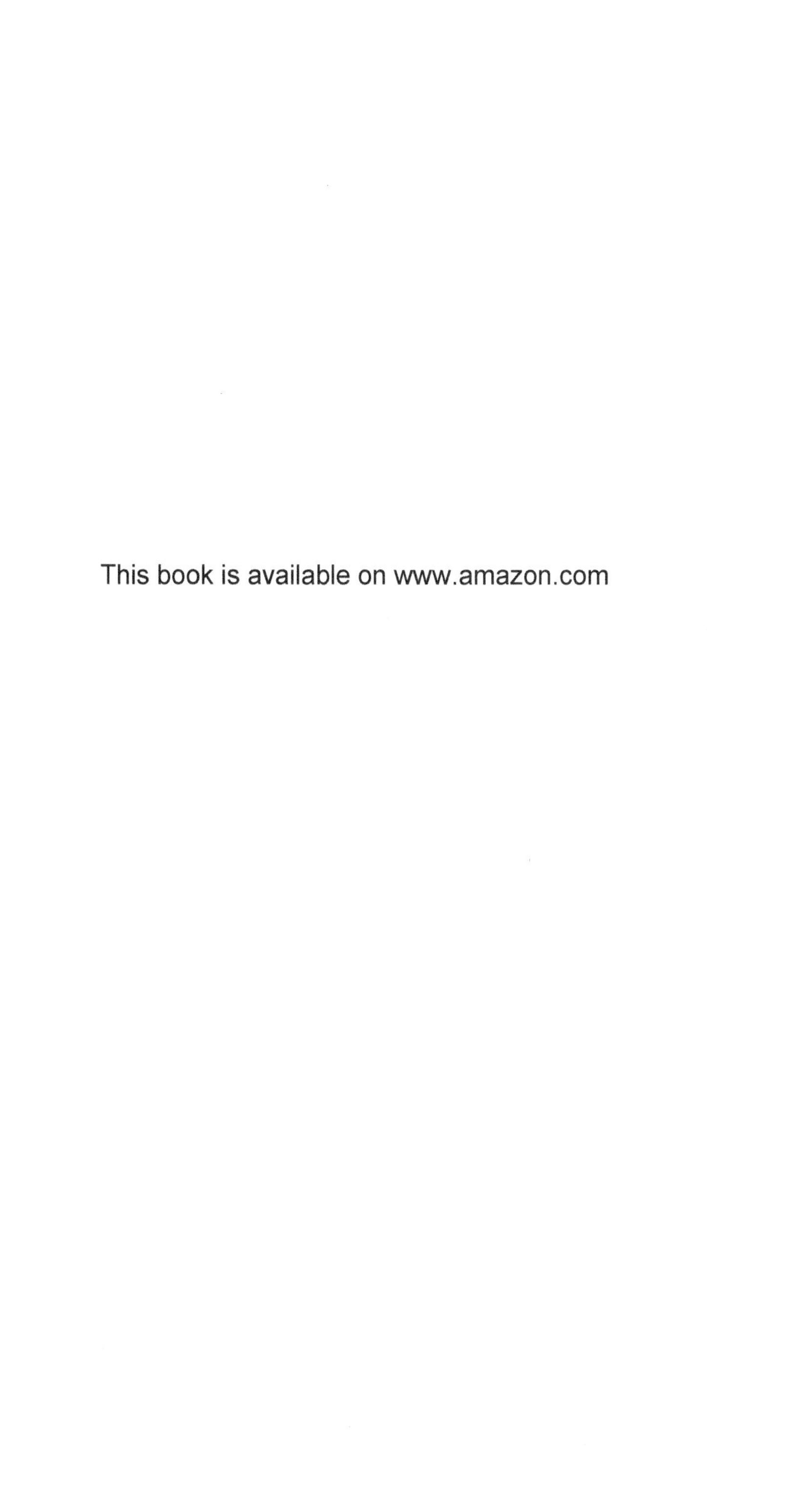